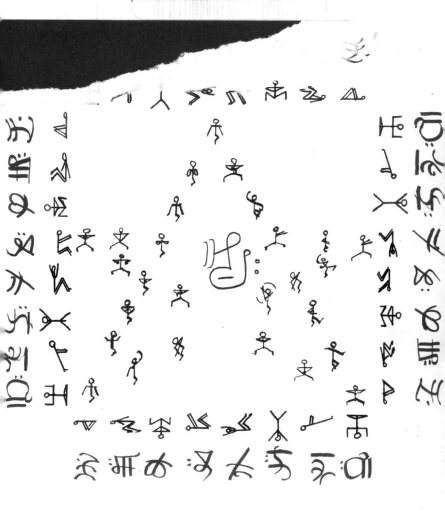

Kum Nye

Kum Nye

Waking Up for Beginners

STEPHANIE WRIGHT

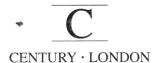

CENTURY · LONDON

Published by Century in 2004

1 3 5 7 9 10 8 6 4 2

First published in the United Kingdom in 2004 by Century
The Random House Group Limited
20 Vauxhall Bridge Road, London SW1V 2SA

Random House Australia (Pty) Limited
20 Alfred Street, Milsons Point, Sydney,
New South Wales 2061, Australia

Random House New Zealand Limited
18 Poland Road, Glenfield,
Auckland 10, New Zealand

Random House South Africa (Pty) Limited
Endulini, 5a Jubilee Road, Parktown 2193, South Africa

The Random House Group Limited Reg. No. 954009
www.randomhouse.co.uk

A CIP catalogue record for this book is available
from the British Library

Papers used by Random house are natural, recyclable products made from
wood grown in sustainable forests. Thr manufacturing processes conform to
the environmental regulations of the country of origin.

ISBN 1 8441 3011 8

Typeset by Palimpsest Book Production Limited,
Polmont, Stirlingshire
Printed and bound in Great Britain by
Clowes Ltd, Beccles, Suffolk

Photographs by Heidie Lee Locke

www.heidieleelocke.com

Dedicated to the family of the
Bön Island of Wickaninnish B.C.
and all its special inhabitants.

CONTENTS

ACKNOWLEDGEMENTS

This introduction to the ancient teaching of Kum Nye has been made possible through the permission and encouragement of my teacher, Christopher Hansard. His support and guidance is integral in the passing on of this knowledge. I thank him for entrusting me with the teachings. I give honour to my teacher, Christopher Hansard, to his teacher, Urgyen Namchuck and to the Lords of the twelve ways of Jangter Bön.

A special thanks to Mari Ryalen for her willingness to model the positions. Thanks also go to David Blount-Porter, Ellen Morton and Anne-Louise Frisby for their generous contributions regarding their experiences. And to my agent Kay McCauley and editor Hannah Black for their constant support and patience throughout the writing of this book.

Within the varied traditions of Tibetan spirituality, both Buddhism and Bön, there have developed many different forms of Kum Nye.

The one presented in this book comes from the Northern Treasure School (Jangter Bön) of the pre-Buddhist Bön culture of ancient Tibet.

This form of Kum Nye is the oldest and can be used in its simplest physical form to benefit your immediate health; in its higher aspects it is a life-changing tool for spiritual development.

In this book, Stephanie Wright, who learnt the

complete system in eight years, brings the simplest physical dimension of Bön Kum Nye to the West for the very first time. The eight exercises will bring you health, the healing of illness, mental clarity and the ability to overcome obstacles.

So it gives me great pleasure to state that this book is an accessible first step to discovering this ancient system of health and vitality. Stephanie Wright's book on this form of Bön Kum Nye has been born out of her own hard training and spiritual development. This book will bring its readers comfort, health and joy.

Christopher Hansard, March 2003
Master Physician of Tibetan Medicine in the Jangter Bön tradition
Medical Director, Eden Medical Centre, Chelsea, London
Author of *The Tibetan Art of Living* and *The Tibetan Art of Positive Thinking*

This book is an introduction to a unique exercise system. It will reveal to you a tool that, when performed as outlined, can bring inumerable benefits. Kum Nye (pronounced *koom neay*) is an amazing life-enhancing regime that offers a fresh approach to health and vitality. With just eight positions you are able to achieve a complete body, mind and spirit workout that takes less than twenty minutes to perform.

Kum Nye can be used by anyone, regardless

of age or fitness. The positive effects of the positions go beyond the physical changes that you will notice. Your energy levels will increase, as will your focus and clarity of thought. Kum Nye is about personal empowerment, it is about cultivating the spirit and enhancing your vitality, it is about unleashing your true potential.

Traditionally taught and passed on as part of an oral teaching, Kum Nye originates from the Tibetan *Dur Bön* tradition, the pre-Buddhist culture of Tibet. As a physical discipline it was taught as a means of survival in an all too hostile environment. Equipping warriors with the threefold tools of strength, endurance and focus for the mind, body and spirit, Kum Nye produced a formidable opponent.

The benefits of Kum Nye were so diverse they became incorporated into other areas of the Dur Bön tradition. Whether your path was that of a soldier, mystic, shaman, astrologer, doctor, yogi or farmer, Kum Nye became part of the foundation teachings. The effects of such a simple set of exercises were hard to ignore.

Today, Kum Nye can be used to enhance your quality of life, enabling you to experience your intrinsic power, increase your vitality and expand your awareness of the natural world around you.

Some versions of Kum Nye as practised in various Buddhist and Bonpo sects are already known in the West. It was not until Buddhism was introduced into Tibet that Kum Nye was integrated into their own practices. The profound positive effects of the exercises are able to enhance awareness, focus and mental clarity, all of which are key steps to achieving enlightenment. To the accomplished student of Kum

Nye, advanced practices of the higher teachings can open doors to spiritual pathways.

This book is the first written introduction to the West of the original Kum Nye from the ancient Dur Bön teachings.

On a daily basis, Kum Nye can be practised as a twenty-minute complete workout, quickly improving your general level of fitness as well as toning and contouring your physique. Postural aches and weaknesses diminish as your muscle tone and body awareness improves. Old injuries can begin to heal and chronic aches and pains diminish. Energy levels are increased and your overall health and vitality improves day by day.

When practised safely within the guidelines of this book, this regular morning routine can give you all you need to face the modern pressures and demands of daily life confidently and positively.

As Kum Nye is a morning exercise regime it helps to regulate the body's metabolic cycles into night and day patterns. This is useful for people who regularly travel long distance. Instead of trying to overcome jetlag while acclimatising and/or attending a bombardment of meetings, twenty minutes of Kum Nye can help reset your body clock.

A contraindication for doing Kum Nye is in the later stages of pregnancy. Do not attempt to perform Kum Nye from the second trimester of pregnancy.

For people with hectic lifestyles and little time for themselves, or those recovering from debilitating illnesses, this quick yet challenging morning routine can give you a thorough workout without having to reach for your gym shoes.

Regardless of the type of exercise or sport you perform as a hobby, Kum Nye can help improve your potential performance in that area. Your inherent level of fitness increases as does your stamina and flexibility, providing your body with an added advantage.

Because of the specific type of energetic dynamics that Kum Nye sets up, it is strongly advised that to receive the maximum benefit from these exercises you attempt to perform them as they have been described in the following chapters. As with many forms of exercise, unless they are done carefully or under supervision there is a chance of injury. To minimise any potential problems, please follow the guidelines and learn the positions slowly rather than all at once. It is strongly advised that none of the positions are used individually for any extended length of time, or used in combination with other forms of exercise systems. If you want to practise other types of exercise that contain an energetic element, for example other Eastern systems like yoga or other styles of Kum Nye, it is suggested you choose a different time of day to practise them. This will enable you to experience the full benefits of Kum Nye and decrease the chances of any unnecessary physical strain or energetic imbalance.

Background

I was brought up in New Zealand within a conservative Western medically influenced background. I decided from a young age that I wanted to help people but without supplying them with countless numbers of pills. I was attracted to the idea of Chiropractic which offered an alternative approach to health and healing and in the early 1980s I made my way to Melbourne, Australia, to study. It is a fascinating profession for its diversity of techniques and approach to health. I spent five years working as a locum in a wide range of clinics, observing various methodologies and applications all suited to the individual practitioner for the benefit of their patients.

After moving to London in the early 1990s, it was not long before I came to the door of the Eden Medical Centre, initially looking for rooms to rent. It was there, while building my Chiropractic practice, that the Principal of the clinic, a master physician of Tibetan medicine,

Christopher Hansard, began to teach a group of students the foundations of Tibetan Dur Bön medicine.

In accordance to tradition, Kum Nye was part of the core teachings given to the novices of this system of medicine. Alongside various other spiritual practices and morning lectures we performed these ancient ways amongst the cobblestones of a London mews.

With my background in anatomy, physiology, sciences and Western exercises it was a challenge to understand the ideology behind such a set of exercises; they were so contradictory to the Western approach to exercise, rehabilitation and musculo-skeletal repair. However, by observing and experiencing this Eastern methodology in action, I have come to appreciate how it challenges the most intrinsic fibres of your being, re-educating your nervous system to work more effectively, relieving the body of old postural habits and pain patterns and providing energy to allow your body to work more efficiently.

Like so many people, over the years my exercise pattern was all or nothing. After the slothful student years, aerobic fever set in. After ten years of dodging sweaty armpits (I'm quite short!) and flailing appendages I hung up my sweat bands and pushed the trainers to the back of the closet. I was tired of the repetition of gym work and a hectic work schedule meant I no longer had a couple of hours free to get to the gym every other day.

I continued on just with my Kum Nye and to my delight I discovered I did not return to my previous pre-aerobics apathy, but continued to be invigorated, energetic and toned. Now, if I do undertake any other form of exercise I don't suffer the usual aches and pains of a new sport and my recovery rate is relatively painless.

Now it is time for you to experience and prosper from the many benefits that this ancient practice can provide.

CHAPTER 1

Calm Abiding

Good morning. Welcome to the dawn of another day.

Each day contains endless possibilities, experiences and sensations just waiting to be appreciated, but only if we are willing and open to see and acknowledge them.

It is easy to wake up, befuddled from a night's dreaming, stumble forth into a day's routine via the remote-controlled breakfast bar and pre-selected mode of transport, to find yourself working on auto-pilot, not quite aware of how you actually got there. Or to awake frantic, panicking and flustered, unable to catch your breath, being propelled manically forward until you collapse, exhausted and overwrought, at the end of the day.

By creating a space for morning calm you can achieve an ongoing balance that allows you to *experience* the day rather than be overruled by it. Even a bad night's rest can be counterbalanced.

Instead of ticking off the days, weeks and months until the next holiday or change of routine, each day can be filled with awakenings, insights and prosperity as you begin to take charge.

As your mind, body and spirit become stronger and more balanced your desires, dreams and limitations alter. Your potential to utilise the tools that you have been born with grows. Clarity of thought overrides confusion and indecision. Vitality and health abound, giving you energy to live life with ease and grace. To experience the natural world around you connects you to who you really are, your inner truth begins to blossom.

Whatever your day has in store for you, being physically, mentally and spiritually prepared can help you overcome any obstacle, rise above any pitfall and learn from any experience. It is not only the big events in life that cause problems but the niggly little recurring annoyances that create stress as well. By being able to set up your day in a calm and harmonious manner, life's little hiccups remain just that instead of developing into full-blown indigestion with a few ulcers on top.

Getting Started

When you first begin to learn these positions start slowly, practising each position for at least a week before you move on to learn the next. This allows you get used to a position and feel confident with it. Because each builds on the other it is important you do not skip a position that you think is too difficult. Persevere as long as you can, then move on to the next. This may mean you could be spending as little as two minutes each morning for the first week.

DO NOT ATTEMPT TO DO ALL THE KUM NYE POSITIONS ON THE FIRST DAY! This is of no advantage and could cause undue stress on your body that will undermine what you are trying to achieve. Take time to learn this discipline and have a little patience. After all, you are learning both to position yourself in a new way and breathe in a new pattern.

The Kum Nye is designed to flow from one position to the next. It is not advisable to change the order or leave out any position if it proves too challenging. And once you have learnt each position there is no advantage to be gained from practising one position on its own – they all build on each other. For the true benefits of Kum Nye, follow the positions in sequence. To begin with you may not be able to perform certain positions perfectly. That is fine. The benefits are still gained by attempting to do them to the best of your ability. Each time you perform them and strive to do them correctly your mind, body and spirit respond. If you have difficulty with a position, do the best you can and then move on to the next. As you persevere it will start to become easier. To get the most out of the exercises you should aim to practise them each morning.

These are incredibly stimulating exercises and if practised in the evening they will upset your body's natural cycles and disturb your sleep patterns. Kum Nye should only ever be performed in the morning.

As you arise, rehydrate yourself with water or a non-caffeinated herbal tea and sit down comfortably in a quiet space big enough to lie down in. Kum Nye can be thirsty work so have plenty of water near you. These exercises can be quite tough so wear clothes you can move in, as light as possible, and bare feet. The exercises produce a lot of body heat and get the circulation flowing throughout your entire system so you should warm up quite quickly. It is not advisable to eat before these exercises as it can put too much pressure on the gut and become uncomfortable.

Create a space that has no distractions. Turn the phones down and occupy the children and animals. This is *your* time of calm. Distractions are curious things of your own making. Something can only distract you if you allow it to. Kum Nye can be performed in the middle of Heathrow Airport at the beginning of the Christmas holiday season with perfect calm, but let us start somewhere a little easier. Turn off the radio and TV. The normal environmental sounds around you are all the sounds you need.

Kum Nye breath pattern

Become aware of how you breathe. Focus on your breath pattern for a few moments and you will instantly notice it changes. Surprising isn't it, how we can go through life without being aware of how we are breathing? Only when something startles us, with our sense of mortality being reawakened, do we notice our breath. Danger, fear, excitement, anticipation, shock, illness, exertion, all of these make us aware that we breathe. By being aware and conscious of how you breathe you connect to your own sense of vitality and mortality as your attention is drawn to the physical. When you regulate your breathing, you can begin to regulate your body and balance other body functions. You begin to become more centred and will notice where you hold tension and where you can relax. As you observe your breath patterns you can begin to understand how they are connected to your thought patterns. Do you hold

19

your breath or sigh a lot? Are your breaths shallow or do you forget to breathe in? What are you thinking or experiencing when this happens?

Try letting go of everything and focusing solely on your breath. Let all your anxieties and fears dissolve. At this time they are of no value and only serve to distract you from something of true importance – living and breathing. Pretty basic stuff, one would think, but so many of us don't create the time to live and breathe. We are too busy just trying to exist. Somewhere along the line of our advancement as a society we forgot the basics.

The breath pattern throughout the Kum Nye is in through the nose and out through the mouth. Practise a few breaths before you begin. Visualise the breath flowing down the centre of your torso and out through your mouth. This will become easier to perform the more you practise, the breath will flow of its own accord.

Each morning, by sitting calmly and still you can begin to gather your thoughts and harness new insights. Your true potential can start to shine through. Dreams you had not realised can become reality. This does not happen overnight but can come a little closer every morning. So here is how you can begin . . .

Position 1

This first position creates a centre of calm, it brings an awareness of space within you and how how expansive you can become. By following your breathing your mind has a chance to slow down and focus, allowing you to become calm and clear. Physically, this position is helpful for neck and shoulder problems. People who are tight across the shoulders, for example due to desk work, or have tension across the chest area either because of pathology or posture, will find this position helpful in stretching out and opening up the upper chest area and shoulder girdle. The postural spinal muscles are stimulated to help you sit upright. Any weakness or imbalance of the spinal musculature will be improved by this position. Hip, pelvic and lower back flexibility will also improve in this position as you sit upright in a cross-legged position. Initially, Calm Abiding will challenge these restricted areas. If they become too uncomfortable, hold the position only for as long as you can, increasing your time by an extra breath each day. There is no rush to do these exercises. Just do them as well as you can each morning.

Practice

Sit down cross-legged. If this position is a problem for you, place a small hand towel, rolled up, at the base of your spine to support your lower back so that you are sitting up as straight as possible. As you persevere with the exercises things like this will become easier.

Raise your left arm out to the side to shoulder height, bend the elbow to bring the forearm and hand to a vertical position, pointing straight upwards and with the palm facing towards your head. Relax your shoulder but keep the elbow at shoulder height. Now, raise the right arm into the same position. Keeping your head straight ahead, and your eyes closed, breathe in through your nose and out through your mouth . . .

This is the first position. Focus on your breath

———

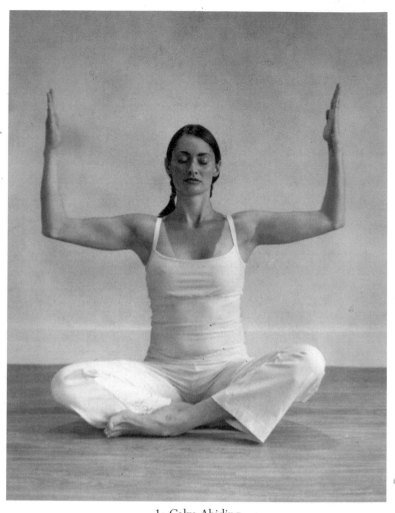

1: Calm Abiding

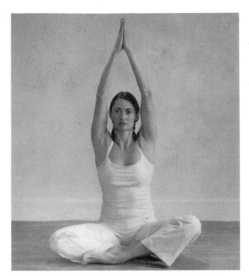

Transition pose

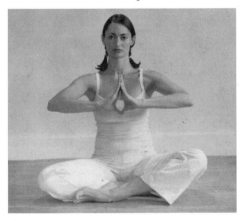

Transition pose

and keeping your arms level. Keep your breath as slow as possible, deep and regular. Build your time gradually up to two minutes. Two minutes is long enough to stay in any of the positions. Even if you feel you can do longer, just rest, there is plenty more to come.

To time yourself you can use a clock until you become able to judge how long two minutes is, or you may choose to measure the time by the number of breaths you take. I suggest to my students that they aim for breathing at a rate of nine breaths in two minutes. These are deep, slow breaths which should be kept at the same rate throughout the eight postures.

In all positions, keep your shoulders down and as relaxed as possible while trying to elongate your neck. If you have had shoulder problems or upper limb complaints this position will help to strengthen previously damaged tissue. Tense neck and shoulders, caused by prolonged computer work, will be stretched and worked to improve the strength, tone and posture and prevent the problem recurring.

Just remember to breathe, slowly and rhythmically in through your nose and out through your mouth. This is the only position performed with your eyes closed, but stay aware of your arm position and peek at the time occasionally until you are sure of your breath count.

Once your two minutes is up, slowly open your eyes and raise your arms up above your head bringing your hands together. Move them down to your chest in a prayer position in preparation for the next position.

CHAPTER 2

Lion's Roar

In this position we continue to work on strengthening and lengthening the spinal postural muscles that were warmed up in Position 1. The
arms, chest and abdominal muscles are also used
in this exercise to support the lower back. This
ensures the entire torso is exercised in Position 2.
On beginning this position most people feel tension across the lower back area. If you have had
previous back problems try this position briefly,
building up your time slowly.

The cardio-vascular system is also worked on

as the heart rate increases while you regulate your breath flow.

Lion's Roar is a position that lends courage, and brings fearlessness in undertaking life's constant challenges.

If you are still a little sleepy then this position will almost certainly revive you. The transition from 1 to 2 should flow gently with one breath in and out. This will become easier as your flexibility improves with practice.

Transition

Once you have completed Calm Abiding, opened your eyes and brought your hands together at your chest, roll your body forwards from the cross-legged position, sliding your hands along the floor in front of you until you are lying on

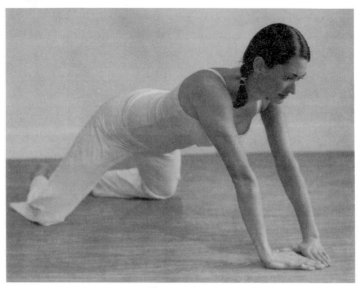

Transition pose

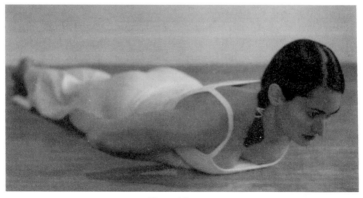

Transition pose

your stomach, your legs stretched out behind you. Make a diamond shape with your hands under your chest – thumbs touching at the base and index fingers at the apex. The feet and toes are pointed. For men, place the left foot over the right so the top of the left foot rests on the sole of the right. For women it is the reverse, with the right foot over the left. This is necessary because of the difference in the direction of flow of energetic pathways between men and women.

Breathe, as with all the positions, in through the nose and out through the mouth. However, this time place your tongue on the roof of your mouth and keep your mouth open the whole time. This also connects energetic pathways flowing throughout your body.

———

Position 2

Now that you have aligned yourself, lift up into Position 2 by straightening your arms – as with a push-up – lifting your torso and both legs off the ground (knees as well) while supporting your weight on the lower foot. Slightly raise your head so your gaze is on the floor a few feet in front of you and your neck is relaxed. Don't forget to breathe!

To protect the lower back make sure your arms are in line with your shoulders directly above your wrists. This gives you the best leverage. If your hands are too far forward or too low it is more difficult to get the leverage to lift and this increases the pressure on your lower back. The golden rule is to place your hands level with your heart.

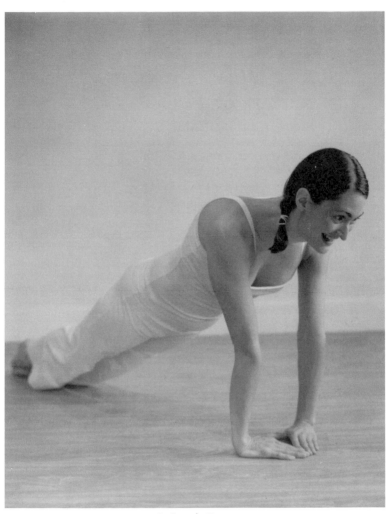

2: Lion's Roar

If you find you are slipping backwards with your feet, point through your feet and lift your body up a little higher.

This position requires confidence and people are often a little nervous when they first start, but it is not as difficult as it first sounds. To be able to maintain the position correct breathing is vital. Remember, one extra breath per day. Breathe all the way down your torso and back out, slowly and deeply. Breathing out through an open mouth will be a little noisy, not quite a lion's roar yet but getting prepared for one. Just imagine coming across an army of Tibetan warriors all practising this position – a formidable sight to behold no doubt!

Again, the aim is to hold this position for up to two minutes. Strength will develop over time. Focusing on the breath will help you endure the position and courage will help you overcome any doubts or fears about maintaining the position.

Once you learn to hold this, it produces great upper body strength, lower back and stomach tone, regulates cardio-vascular activity and increases lung capacity. This all helps to improve your general level of fitness.

Exercises are regularly used in Western medicine to rehabilitate the body after injury or trauma. Various active and passive stretching techniques are used as well as general fitness exercises such as walking, cycling and swimming. Kum Nye incorporates stretching and muscle contracting methods but predominantly relies on resistance stretching and isometric contractions where the muscles do not shorten during contraction. Here joints, ligaments, joint capsules and tendons and the vital fluids are exerted beyond the normal range of everyday use. This produces a more supple yet strong body which will improve both flexibility and endurance as well as lower the risk of other potential sporting injury.

Old injuries or traumas can sometimes resurface while performing Kum Nye and chronic conditions can flare up. This is not a bad thing and if done slowly and correctly, Kum Nye can help your body repair these conditions. For example, it is not uncommon for an old fracture to start to ache or a shoulder previously injured to become restricted within its range of movement once again. This is temporary, it does not last. Keep practising the Kum Nye and these symptoms will pass within a few weeks leaving the areas stronger and healthier than before.

In the Tibetan Bön tradition it is taught that muscles hold the memory of everything your body has experienced. The breath pattern, working with the positions, helps to release those negative experiences produced by illness or trauma that hinder complete physical, emotional and spiritual recovery.

Chronic back pain usually has a large emotional component to it. Years of constant, recurrent pain causes a depression of the mind, body and spirit. Physical therapies often provide only temporary relief. Even surgery can be unsuccessful in eliminating pain and dysfunction. Each time the symptoms recur the emotional impact is reinforced. Kum Nye — and particularly this position — will challenge a weakened back. It may even feel as if it is exacerbating the problem. But do have courage; each day try to do a little more. Slowly and surely it will strengthen and repair the weakened areas as well as helping you overcome the emotional responses to the condition.

The Tibetan Bön medical system teaches that the spine is the largest emotional organ in the body. Everything you feel and experience is related back through the spine and up to the brain. Everything you do passes through and impacts on the spine. An injury to any area of the body will have an effect on the spinal function, influencing the way you respond and relate to yourself, everyone and everything around you. This experience can be expressed in a multitude of forms, from physical pain and dysfunction to visceral dysfunction and emotional releases.

Your spine holds the key to an integrated well-being. As you practise Kum Nye you will begin

———

to develop emotional stability, spiritual insight and your structural alignment will improve. Just continue to persist slowly and gently with this position (and indeed all of the positions). Some days will be better than others yet this does not mean that one day is less effective than the other. When you consciously give up or sabotage yourself with thoughts like 'I can't, I can't', don't fret. The act of persisting every day will bring benefits. Change those negative mantras for more positive and affirming ones: 'I can, I can' or 'I have, I have'. Each day the Kum Nye is going to be different. Some days a position is a breeze, and the day after that it's like you've never done it before. I cannot stress enough that by persisting to the best of your ability each day, your strength, endurance and focus will increase, bringing benefits to all aspects of your life.

———

Because of the integrated nature of this exercise system, it will have a positive impact on any other type of exercise you choose to do. If Kum Nye is the only form of exercise you do, it will naturally improve your general level of fitness, strength, endurance and focus. When combined with other types of exercise, the discipline will further increase stamina, flexibility and concentration thus improving your performance and enjoyment as well as limiting the potential for injury. There are no physical exercises that are inappropriate to practise with Kum Nye. However, if you practise Eastern systems such as yoga, where specific breathing techniques are applied and energetic pathways are activated, you will find the energetic nature of Kum Nye will become the more dominant force. Some people experience emotional outburst as a side effect of performing Western exercises that involve controlled breathing techniques such as Pilates. The system of Kum Nye created thousands of years ago was designed to produce specific energetic reactions within the individual and the emotional release is regarded as an integral part of the system. This book introduces you to this ancient system of knowledge for the first time.

Breathe deeply and prepare yourself for the next position.

CHAPTER 3

Connecting Heaven and Earth

Now it is time to move out of Lion's Roar and into the third position. This position concentrates on the torso – toning and strengthening the abdominal muscles, stretching and expanding the chest cavity as well as improving the function of the gut.

Some beginners have mentioned that they experience nausea while performing this position. Depending on the situation, this may be due either to an emotional factor or a physiological reaction caused by excitation of the vagus nerve. Whatever the trigger, the nausea will pass in its own time. In Tibetan Bön terms this clearing of blockages is considered a 'good' sign, but if you do experience anything like this just slow down and breathe as slowly and deeply as you can. Pause and take some water before you move on.

Practice

From Position 2, unfold your feet and carefully walk your hands back towards them, keeping your knees as straight as possible, and then stand up. Now, take a step out to the side with either foot so you are standing with your feet positioned slightly wider than your shoulders with your feet facing forward. Lift both arms above your head, reaching upwards to the sky, palms

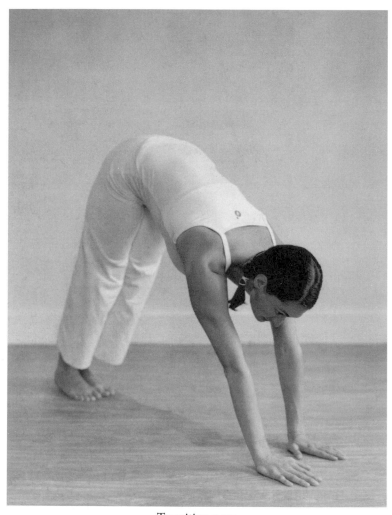

Transition pose

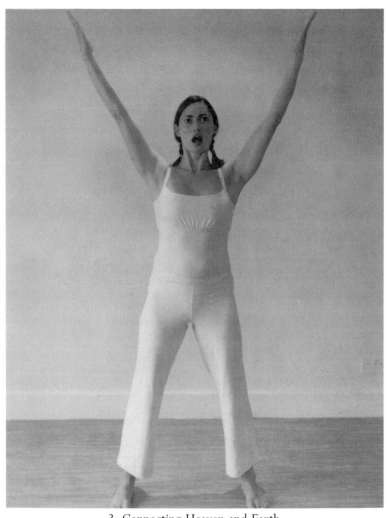

3: Connecting Heaven and Earth

facing inwards, shoulders down and relaxed. Have your mouth open as wide as you can while you inhale and exhale but with your tongue relaxed this time. You are still breathing in through your nose and out through your mouth. Look up and tilt your head slightly backwards. Lengthen your neck by keeping your shoulders relaxed. Keep your knees straight and push into the ground with your feet. Breathe slowly and deeply, exhaling noisily. Imagine you are stretching upwards to reach the sky whilst pushing your feet down into the earth, expanding the space in between. Allow your stomach to relax and expand rather than tensing it and holding it in.

This stretching and expansion of your torso makes more space for your digestive system and will assist the intestinal function. The thoracic diaphragm is lifted upwards with the rise of the arms while the pelvic organs are pushed a little lower. This creates more space for the intestines to rumble through. The more relaxed and toned the intestines, the better the absorption and elimination processes will function. Yawning and burping in this position is a good sign! This indicates that trapped gas is moving out and releasing blockages within the digestive tract. Stomach exercises, like sit-ups, contract and restrict the gut causing tension and constriction; this can aggravate it and cause dysfunction. This alternative method strengthens and tones the abdominal muscles and helps to produce a more defined muscular torso. This is achieved by the combination of positions, and not due to one specific position.

This pose is not passive. The abdominal

muscles gain strength by being exercised in this isometric manner. Try and focus on lengthening the torso while breathing correctly.

It can be very liberating standing wide with your mouth open, torso exposed, neck out-stretched. Having your throat open and exposed in this manner can unleash emotional blocks that may have suppressed self-expression. I found this position emotionally challenging when I first began. Even in the privacy of my own home I felt very exposed. Then, after a few months, this was replaced with a sense of liberation and con-nectedness. Finding your own voice is powerful medicine. The neck is the essential link between the mind and body. To connect clearly the neck must be as open and flowing as possible.

The first three positions work primarily on the

upper body. The neck, shoulders and chest are the main focus of attention. Therefore the muscle groups that tone up the quickest are the upper arms – triceps and biceps – trapezius, deltoid and the pectoral muscles of the chest. The abdominal muscles are also quick to respond. Many pleasantly surprised women students in my class remark how their bust line improves, while the men comment on the definition of their abdominals. Shoulders start to become broader as the postural muscles of the spine begin to strengthen and people stand taller with ease.

This change in physique continues to improve as we move to the other positions and involve the lower limbs more, thus developing tone and strength in the buttock, thighs, legs and feet. This is not a fat-burning exercise or a cellulite buster as such, but it does change your metabolism and help with lymphatic flow and blood supply to all areas of the body as well as toning all the muscle groups at once, giving an overall workout. Body shapes begin to change. Of course this is influenced by whatever genetics you have been blessed with but in general women tend to become more curvaceous (in the right places) while men begin to develop the defined triangle shape – broad shoulders and toned midriff – or a more powerful rectangular shape. Physiologically, this is a response to the muscle groups working in unison.

The Kum Nye will also begin to make you aware of how you operate within your environment, when and in what situations particular responses occur, how you react and the emotion that is connected to it. Old adages like 'that person is a pain in the neck!' are based on truth. Sometimes our body reacts to someone or something without us really noticing. Shoulders may tense, jaws clench and before we know it our neck seizes up. As you become more aware of how you are reacting to certain situations or people, you begin to operate within your environment in a less reactive manner. This reduces the amount of unnecessary and potentially damaging tension you carry around with you on a regular basis.

Kum Nye changes your physical shape to fit the physiological, emotional and energetic potential that you have. Some people find their appetite is stimulated when they first start, others find it decreases. Once again this balances in its own time to find a comfortable medium. If someone has had a restricted range of food types and flavours in their diet they may experience a desire for specific or atypical flavours and food. One entrapment is, of course, chocolate. This food is often craved initially because in Tibetan classification of food types chocolate contains all the flavours that our palate is accustomed to, therefore supplying an instant hit of whatever your body craves. All food can be used as medicine in Bön terms, however, everything in moderation!

The three humours

There are three underlying energetic forces that govern the mind, body and spirit. These are called the three humours: wind, bile and phlegm. The three humours are the dynamic forces that exist within every level of our body, mind and spirit. Every thought, action, cell, organ, interconnection and interaction between ourselves and the world around us, intellectually, emotionally and spiritually are governed by our humours.

While we are all made up of the three humours there is usually one that will be dominant. The particular combination will influence your body shape, what type of foods you are attracted to, how you eat them and what foods you can use as medicine for yourself. The various humeral compositions create characteristic body shapes which the Kum Nye will help to encourage, as well as allowing all three humours to interact in a way that is unique to us individually. The Kum Nye works in a psychosomatic manner to bring the humours into balance.

———

There are many factors involved regarding our body shapes and types, but the following will give an overall idea. Wind-dominant people are classically bony and angular-looking with lithe, strong, supple bodies. Bile types are active, with good endurance. Phlegm-dominant people are prone to holding weight especially when emotionally upset, but they have a robust constitution. The combinations possible allow for personal variations of course. It is also possible to rebalance the humours, which will instigate changes in the body's shape. Kum Nye and dietary changes are just two ways this can be achieved within the vast range of tools and techniques used in Tibetan medicine.

CHAPTER 4

Flying Drum

The upper torso has by now had a pretty good stretch. Now you are ready to assume and begin Flying Drum.

Position 4 is particularly good for strengthening and toning the buttocks, thighs and lower legs. It also begins to work on the numerous muscles that support the feet. Focusing on your breath is important as it will help you to maintain your balance in this position.

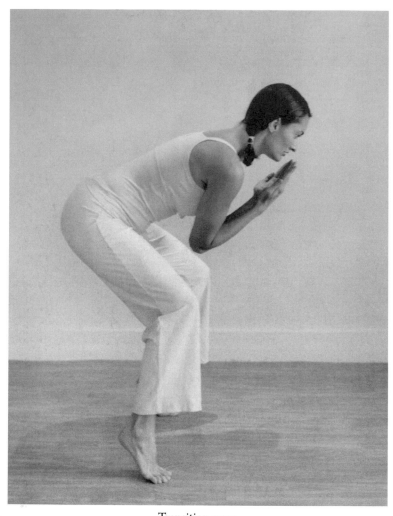

Transition pose

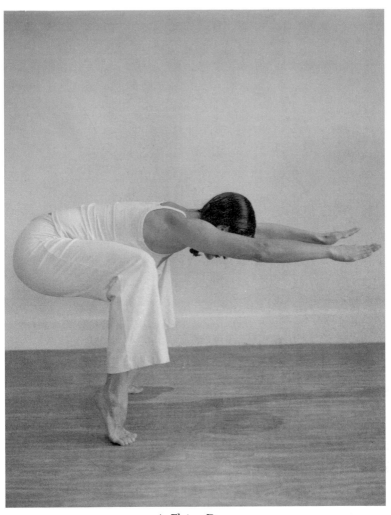

4: Flying Drum

Practice

Leave your feet at the width you established in Position 3. Bring your arms down in front of you while you crouch down and lean forwards, bending your hips and knees and stand on the balls of your feet. Stretch your arms forward in front of you, palms facing downwards, keeping your shoulders relaxed and your neck long. Fix your gaze towards the ground slightly in front of you. Your back should be as flat and level as you can get it. Push your knees outwards to help balance and squeeze the calves tightly, this will help to stop any shaking in the leg muscles that sometimes develops. Your mouth is no longer opened wide as in the previous two poses; relax it and breathe in through your nose and out through your mouth. Once again the breath is the key to maintaining this position.

This position is usually felt very quickly in the thighs as a deep burning stretch but try to keep going for as long as you can, increasing your time slowly. This position is great for anyone who fancies a spot of skiing. Flying Drum will strengthen the quadriceps and calf muscles. It will also help any weaknesses of the feet and ankles, for example fallen arches and weak ligaments. If you have experienced previous knee, ankle or hip trauma start this exercise carefully and slowly. You may experience discomfort in old injury sites but these will be temporary and the more you persevere the stronger the tissues will become. This may feel quite disconcerting for some people but, as explained in Chapter 2, in Tibetan medicine this is described as the release of the 'memory' that remains imprinted in your nervous system, in a physical form, of the trauma that is still held in the tissues which may prevent them achieving complete recovery or predispose them to degenerative changes in the future.

While taking classes I find there are a few recurring questions and experiences that my students tend to raise. They often remark that their dreams become more vivid or intense. They may have better recall or even start lucid dreaming. In this Bön tradition it is believed that your muscles hold the memory of past events in picture form. While you are asleep these images can be expressed and processed within the nervous system in dream form. Kum Nye works on the muscles in a particular way that encourages the release of past traumas or accidents as well as activating the nervous system to operate more efficiently. As you sleep, the actions of the memory are released from the muscles that have been storing everything you have experienced and reacted to during the day. At night your nervous system has a chance to catalogue and organise the information you have received and processes it into a format you can interpret in the future. This takes place in dream time. If you are inclined to this sort of awareness you will notice an increase in dream recollection. Be assured this is a safe method, your mind will only process what it is ready and able to cope with. This is an intermittent occurrence and is not experienced by everyone. An interesting consequence of this phenomenon is that you may note a change in the holding of your Kum

Nye positions. The emotional shift will change the way your body holds itself and your position will become more aligned. Initially though it may feel even more difficult.

Sometimes disillusion occurs during the latter weeks of the Kum Nye course. When the students begin to practise Positions 5 or 6 there is occasionally a sense of frustration or even defeat, when they feel they are not improving. Of course this is specific to each person but most commonly the challenge is with positions 2 and 5. This vexation is because of a lack of advancement in what they would consider, in Western terms, a decent length of time.

Kum Nye is designed NOT to be mastered in just a physical way, nor in a mind over matter way. Only by the mind, body and spirit being in unison does the Kum Nye become complete.

———

Finding the poses difficult does not mean you are not improving – it is just not in the manner you are accustomed to. What you will notice, even if a position feels as if it is getting harder, is that other benefits will become more apparent, little things like your posture improving, not being too tired to sit or stand correctly and your general level of fitness increasing regardless of how the postures themselves feel. Your reflexes improve and your focus becomes clearer while your body's metabolism becomes more efficient. So persevere and the positions will adjust of their own accord.

A number of people who have attended my courses have histories of debilitating illnesses. For some it was a long time ago and others more recently. Others have experimented with drugs and alcohol. Both cases can result in a deep-seated and insidious debilitation of the body's nervous system, immune system and organ function. When these students begin to do the Kum Nye they often feel a deep fatigue. Although I describe these exercises as invigorating and stimulating, to these people the positions can leave them drained and unmotivated. They can feel very tired and have difficulty getting up in the morning (a great excuse to not do the exercises) as the symptoms mimic their past conditions or hangovers. The Kum Nye is releasing the deep fatigue that is still held within their bodies and causing the detoxification of all the body's systems. By performing the Kum Nye in the mornings, eating a properly balanced diet and avoiding stimulants and excessive sugars, your body will have the best chance to repair itself while you sleep. The fatigue will lift and your body and mind will begin to work in harmony. There are many factors involved in illness and well-being patterns, and each person is unique. But a few simple steps can help everyone begin the road to recovery.

Something else people sometimes notice when they first start is their lowered tolerance for alcohol. This is due to the detoxification effect of the Kum Nye and the way it affects your metabolism. (But, take note, Kum Nye is a great hangover cure!) Similarly, if Kum Nye is performed by people who indulge in social drug-taking, because of the manner in which Kum Nye affects the mind, body and spirit, even casual and intermittent drug usage can induce depressive cycles, emotionally, physically and spiritually. However high the high gets, the low can get lower so it is not recommended that you perform Kum Nye if you use drugs – however infrequently.

As your sense of awareness changes you will begin to see things differently. Some people note that they become more emotional or angry, they become less tolerant with situations they are unhappy with. These experiences are but temporary blips as the mind, body and spirit begin to harmonise. As awareness continues to develop behaviour will become more skilful and the anger is dissipated.

Don't let this deter you and be assured that lots of people feel an immediate sense of calm and lightness when they begin the Kum Nye. Spiritual development is unique to each person.

Some people perceive light or visual alterations when they start Kum Nye, either while performing Kum Nye or during the day. They may experience auras or vibrancy of colours in objects around them. In the same way, some people become aware of their hearing changing. They pick up sounds acutely and become in tune with the natural rhythms and beats surrounding them. For other people it is their intuition that is stimulated. They become more sensitive to what is happening around them, the needs of other people and what is best for their own personal development. Smell can also be enhanced, along with sensitivity to touch.

I am often asked if it is possible to practise one position on its own in order to develop it or if it is possible to skip a position that feels too difficult. The answer to both of these questions is no. Nothing will be gained by practising one position on its own or avoiding a difficult position, as the Kum Nye is a flowing movement. Each position builds on the others before and after it. They become a harmonised unit of power, and missing a position is the equivalent of removing a battery.

I mentioned earlier that Kum Nye can affect the digestive system. After a few weeks of starting the Kum Nye some people may find that their bowel motions increase for a short period of time as the body detoxifies. Think of it as Kum Nye performing 'internal aerobics' on your organ system. This is short-lived and very natural, so there is no need to worry.

Let's move on to the next position . . .

CHAPTER 5

Honour to the Earth King

This is where the word 'burn' is given a whole new meaning.

Because of the intensity of this posture I would recommend that you spend at least two to four weeks practising the first four positions before moving on to this pose. This is a demanding position and the more you prepare for it, the easier the posture will be. You do not have to be able to perform the previous positions perfectly before moving on to the next, however you should be able to move through and hold each position for a few breaths before moving on. There is no need to rush, take as long as necessary to learn each pose.

Practice

Move your hands from the outstretched position of Flying Drum and place them on the ground in front of you. Keep your elbows straight with your hands slightly forward, not directly under your shoulders. Squat down slightly to lower your backside so that it is level with your spine and your spine is parallel to the floor, leave a little gap just wide enough to put your fingers in behind the knee. You are still balancing on the balls of your feet, but the arch is dropped a little and your knees are pushed out-

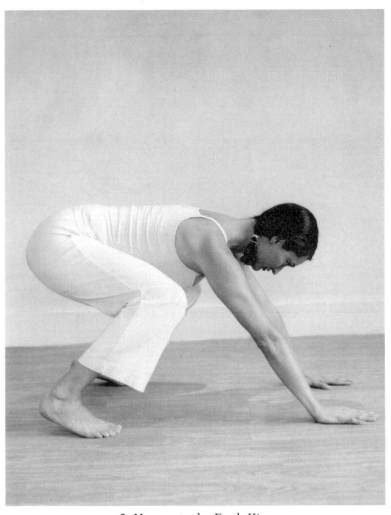

5: Honour to the Earth King

wards. Do not rest the weight of your trunk on your thighs or legs.

Breathe the Kum Nye breath, concentrating on it flowing all the way through your torso and then returning up and out of your mouth. Imagine your breath as a horizontal tube of air travelling one way then reversing back on itself. This column of air becomes like a pole that gives you the strength and support you need to maintain this position.

If you find this position continuously easy then it is unlikely you are doing it correctly.

Position 5 is challenging and demands even more focus to endure the intensity of the workout. Concentrating on the breath will help you transcend any physical discomfort as well as heightening your awareness. Try not to pant, keep your breath slow and regular and

---

remember to keep your eyes open. Once you think you have done as much as you can, take another couple of breaths before stopping.

The cardio-vascular system certainly gets a workout here. When I first started practising this position the burn in my thighs was remarkable, particularly as I was already quite fit. I was cycling daily and performing high-powered aerobics up to six days a week as well as dance classes, yet after a couple of minutes in this position I felt as weak as a kitten. However it was not long before I began to notice that my ability to jump and perform leg raises in class had increased and my reflexes were sharpened. I had been performing various aerobic classes and cross training for five years and my level of fitness had reached a plateau. Then with the Kum

---

Nye it changed. My fitness level shifted up another notch, giving me much more stamina and a much shorter recovery time.

I admit this position proved to be the most challenging for me. For a long time I could not work out how to improve it and the more I tried the more resistant it seemed to be. My fitness continued to improve, but I had formed a mental block about this position. Whereas the other positions fluctuated between good days and tough days, this position remained stubborn. Eventually I realised that until I discovered what the emotional obstruction was that prevented me from proceeding with this pose it would remain difficult. I had to let this unfold in its own time.

This 'time' took four years . . . you can't rush personal development! One morning there was

---

a shift. These shifts happen in all the positions in their own time and are like little 'awakenings', giving you personal insights and realisations as well as producing physical shifts in the way you hold a position. While in Honour to the Earth King the position produced the most intense heat that travelled from my chest down into my arms and hands and beyond. I felt as though my heart had begun to open. My legs were still under exertion but they felt strong and vibrant. The experience was liberating and I was left elated, energised and extremely excited at the realisation of what I had experienced.

Any time the positions become too difficult I go back and listen to my heart. I try to work out what I have done to close up again. I try to send kindness to myself and slowly but surely it begins to ease again.

———

Once you have achieved an awareness it requires nurturing and care to encourage it to continue to flourish and bloom. Keep looking deeper into yourself to see who you are and accept what you are shown. Allow yourself to become wise, joyous and humble.

CHAPTER 6

Honouring the Lineage

Humility is the key to understanding the 'philosophical' nature of this posture. When you crouch low to the ground in the manner described below, the posture encourages an awareness of your own place in the greater scheme of things. It is a position in which to contemplate your origins, where you came from, how you arrived where you are. Physically, this position affects the ankle, knee and hip joints and how they interconnect.

Practice

Roll back into a squatting position. Place your heels down on the ground. If your positioning was correct in Position 3 you should not have to move your feet closer or further apart to adopt the squat. If it is difficult to get your feet flat on the ground your feet are too close. If they are too far apart there is excessive strain placed on the knee joints and you will have a tendency to lean too far forward. Your toes can point forwards or to the side, whatever feels more natural for you. Push your knees outwards so your body can sink lower between them. Bring your hands together in front of you, holding them in a prayer position and keep your forearms touching. Keep your eyes open and breathe, deep and slow. Be aware of your

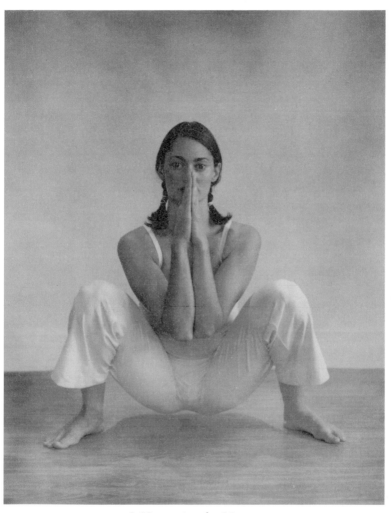

6: Honouring the Lineage

alignment. Check that you are as centred as possible and not favouring one hip. After a period of time you may feel a sigh as your body relaxes into the position. The pelvis sinks down lower and relaxes a little. It becomes a very comfortable position.

This is a peaceful and humble position. For those of you with an emotional disposition this position can release tears. Breathe deeply and gently to find peace and calm if this happens. Feel the breath flowing down to your perineum and back up and out of your mouth. This flow allows the pelvic area to relax. According to Bön beliefs the pelvic area is home to vital life force. For health and vitality this needs to be kept flowing throughout the body. If it is stagnant and restricted we become imbalanced, our immunity weakens and other vital life forces within the body become weakened. One example of this is the role of the fluid in our joints. From a Western viewpoint, synovial fluid is important for the lubrication of the joints and for mobility. Dur Bön teaches that this fluid also contains essential antibodies vital for the overall health of all the body's systems. Proper joint function and range of motion is essential for the maintenance of the whole body. If any joint is restricted it is important to try and regain as much mobility as possible and to keep working the area to maintain as much muscle and ligamentous strength as possible.

When all the supporting components are working as best as they can they will help support any other area of dysfunction in the body. In Tibetan Dur Bön medicine all the body systems are interconnected, integrated and dependent on each other. Vital forces flow throughout the body in channels that pass through and connect organs to muscles, nerves, bone, fat, connective tissue, blood and lymph and other fluids. If one system of the body is not working well it has an impact on the 'whole' body.

We spend a lot of time sitting in cars and chairs. These positions restrict the tissues around the hips and buttocks. Walking is a good general exercise to free up hip restrictions but Kum Nye stretches the joints more extensively.

In this position, the area where the quadriceps (front thigh muscles) and the knee joints meet is placed under maximum strain. Any previous knee injury or instability will be challenged and old symptoms may resurface. All I can say is persevere. Slowly and gently work through the position, it will eventually make the injured tissue stronger. The quadriceps will gain flexibility and the joint stability and strength will improve.

Ankles are considered to be 'sacred' joints in Tibetan medicine. It is taught that they are different to other joints as they contain healing properties within their synovial fluid. When I first began Kum Nye my left ankle would swell up of its own accord. There was no pain or joint restriction, just swelling. I put it down to twisting my ankle a lot as a child when the joints were very unstable. This swelling eventually passed with practise and I am now very sure-footed.

If someone has a lower back or pelvic problem it can manifest itself in the knee joint. This is due to the complex attachments of the thigh muscles to both the hip, pelvis and knee.

Similarly it is possible for there to be restriction in lumbar spine mobility or a pelvic dysfunction with the pain only registering around the knee joint. Old sporting injuries such as hamstring tears can cause a restriction in the pelvic range of motion which can lead to chronic back discomfort. The mechanics of the whole lower body need to be examined as a unit and not as separate parts. The next few positions will help to re-establish proper balance of all the thigh muscles.

When I first started this chapter I thought I would have a lot to say. After all, plenty of my students have experienced knee discomfort. But I got stuck. Really stuck. Then it occurred to me that for the previous few weeks I had been experiencing some pain in my left knee while trying to bend it. I hadn't noticed any discomfort during my practices but that in itself is not unusual. Then I noticed that within a very short space of time I had no less than ten people from various Kum Nye courses coming to me for treatment for knee problems. Some had been Kum Nye-related and others developed from seemingly unrelated incidents. I figured the Universe was trying to teach me something – but I still couldn't work out what! Then I remembered what knees are about. They are about moving forward, progressing through life, walking fearlessly but with humility. It takes great courage to be humble and to let go of the things we think give us meaning and the things we hold to justify our existence. We get frustrated and feel stuck when we are unable to decide where to go, which direction to turn to,

---

what option is the best. Honouring the Lineage offers you an opportunity to find out where you came from, what makes you who you are and how you can cultivate that and grow. To move forwards, humbly yet courageously.

While in this position I occasionally experience spontaneous flashbacks of past events, conversations I have had or a realisation of how I have reacted to some situation. This is part of the Kum Nye experience and is an example of how the mind and body are working together in these positions. The pose, coupled with the breath pattern, can trigger an emotional release. It is not always pleasant. Reminding myself of when I have spoken too abruptly and without considering the consequences, or not appreciating the effect my words can have on someone is very chastening. It may be a misunderstanding I've had with my family, caused by bad habits of communication that have developed over the years. But rather than ignoring these patterns it is better to understand where they stem from and transform them through self-knowledge. This does not happen overnight. It takes practice to catch yourself from falling back into old patterns and habits, but each time you do it gets a little easier. To honour the lineage that I was born from and accept my family's actions, past and present, good and bad, is a humbling experience. The further back into my heritage I go, the more it connects me to all of humanity and I am able to express humility and compassion to all living beings in this manner, not just the nearest and dearest. Practising the Kum Nye every day certainly reinforces the need to keep striving for personal growth as well as physical well-being, to keep moving forward . . .

———

To honour the lineage is also about honouring the traditions that the Kum Nye came from. With all their wisdom and compassion, they created a tool which we can use to transform and heal ourselves and the world around us. A tool that can be used to help us live our lives the best possible way we can, humbly and fearlessly, knowing we have made informed choices to the best of our ability and acted on them accordingly for the benefit of all.

The complexity of these exercises continues to astound me. Just as you feel you have reached a level of understanding, another starts to unfold. With my own permission, the Kum Nye enables me to continue to bloom, physically, mentally and spiritually.

You know, I think my knee feels better already.

CHAPTER 7

Awakening Central Channel

Position 7, Awakening Central Channel, refers to the spinal column and spinal cord. This position will lengthen the spine and neck and improve the function of the spinal nerves as they travel up and down the spine. The hip joints will also be rotated, helping to increase their range of motion and flexibility further. As you strengthen the muscle tone of the pelvic area and increase the suppleness of the supporting joints, the overall health of the body will improve. Again, this is because the Tibetan Bön medical system regards vitality and well-being as dependent on the proper functioning of the pelvic organs, muscles and joints.

Practice

From Position 6 roll backwards to lie down on the floor. Place your arms on the ground by your side, palms down. Relax your neck and shoulders. Bring your knees up towards your chest and turn them outwards towards your shoulders while you raise your lower legs towards the ceiling. Now, flex your feet so the soles are facing the sky.

Traditionally, lit candles were placed on the soles of the feet to make sure they didn't move from the position although hot yak butter dripping down the legs possibly isn't a nice

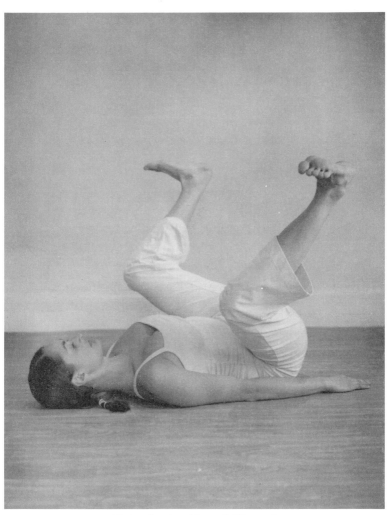

7: Awakening Central Channel

experience. Bear in mind these exercises were traditionally performed in next to nothing, or less. To inspire you to keep the correct position, imagine you too have candles placed on the soles of your feet. This way may prove to be a little less messy!

Breathing in through your nose and out your mouth, feel the breath going all the way down your trunk and back up. Keep your pelvis down on the floor while you try and bring your knees closer to your chest and rotate them outwards at the hip. Breathe, relax and lengthen the spine. This position will help tone the pelvic floor muscles as well as work the hip rotator muscles and ligaments of the hip joint. Some people fall naturally into this position. If one hip appears to turn less than the other, keep trying to rotate it as much as you can. Anyone who has had fractures of the hip, pelvis or thigh, congenital anomalies of the region or disease of the hip (e.g. arthritis) may find there is some restriction in the hip flexibility.

In Position 7 the spine is more restricted than in the previous 6 positions and the pelvis is not weight-bearing. All the work must be done through the rotation of the legs. Avoid the temptation to pull your legs closer to your chest with your hands – this is cheating! Keep working with the thigh muscles and pull your legs closer to your body while you turn your knees out as far as you can.

Because each position has an impact on the other positions, the more flexibility you gain from this position the better the previous ones will get and vice versa.

This stretch uses the weight of your trunk to

elongate the spine while the rotation of the hips pushes the lumbar curve down. This changes the positional tension on the spinal cord itself and by doing so it is believed the mechanics between the cord and the rest of the nervous system are improved. Breath helps the cycle of vitality down through the body to the pelvic region and back up through the organs to the brain. All the components of the central nervous system are getting a workout – stimulating, toning and awakening.

CHAPTER 8

Balance

This is the last position and completes the cycle of Kum Nye. It balances both the physical body by engaging all of the limbs down to the fingers and tocs as well as the energetic cycles of the body, creating equilibrium before you continue with the rest of your day.

This position helps to stretch the spine and the muscles at the back of the arms and legs. If you haven't been putting all of your energy into the previous positions then you'll have to now!

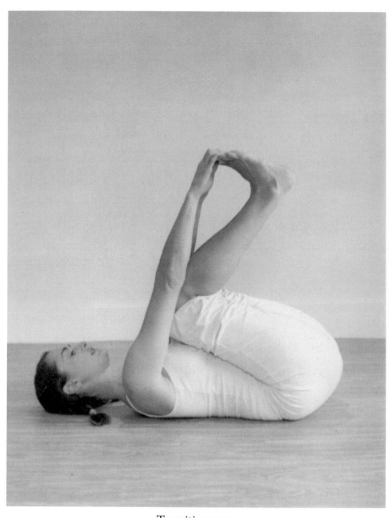

Transition pose

Practice

With your legs still raised, bring your knees together and grasp your toes with your fingers. Keeping your neck and shoulders relaxed on the floor and your bottom on the ground, try and straighten your legs. This is easy enough if you lift your spine off the ground but that is not the position! To get the proper stretch keep your spine and pelvis down. If your knees are bent persist and keep trying to straighten them as much as you can. As you continue to hold your toes and stretch your legs into the air you will be able to straighten your legs a little more with each breath. This is due to a muscle reflex that comes into play, called 'creep'. This occurs in increments but is enough to be noticeable and will improve every time you do the Kum Nye.

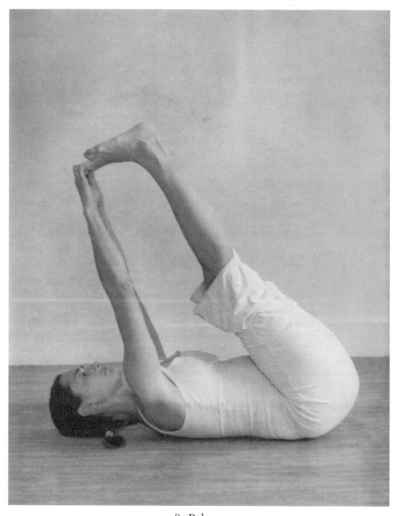

8: Balance

Only by applying this pressure over a period of time do the muscles lengthen. Research has demonstrated that the lengthening of muscles is most effectively achieved by stretching them with low, constant force for prolonged periods of time at elevated temperatures. By now your body temperature should be raised and your muscles supple and ready to stretch as much as they can. It is not only your legs that will be stretched here, but also the arm and spinal muscles. Keep your Kum Nye breath slow and regular to help you focus in this position.

As the name suggests, this position requires balance. Don't worry if you topple over to one side during your initial attempts at straightening your legs, it just shows an imbalance in the tension of the muscles of your spine, pelvis and/or shoulder girdle. As you become stronger, your alignment will adjust and your muscles will rebalance to allow you to become centred again.

As you are pulling your toes down you are flexing your foot which forcibly stretches your Achilles tendon. The Achilles tendon is the largest and strongest tendon in the body and is essential for proper gait and agility. But it requires regular stretching to remain supple and to prevent injury. The foot itself is often over-looked when it comes to stretching and exer-cising the body. The ankle and foot are susceptible to numerous ligamentous and soft tissue injuries as well as stress fractures, either as a by-product of poor exercise technique or a lack of proper exercise. The more controlled a stretch, the more elasticity acquired, the better the function of the foot and ankle.

On an energetic level this position helps

balance the body. As you hold your toes you are creating a cycle of energy that runs through your torso and along your limbs. This is facilitated by your breath.

This position stretches the posterior thigh muscles that have been held in tension during the previous positions. The front thigh muscles that were stretched are now contracted. At the same time the fine intrinsic muscles of the spinal vertebrae are pulled and stretched to give a comprehensive workout. If you are not warm yet I would suggest you have not been breathing properly. Even very fit people will warm up with a decent stretch.

When you stretch muscles that are not used to being exerted in this manner for a prolonged period of time, they begin to shake – not just the fine quivering of a few muscle fibres but enough to make the whole limb shake. This may have already happened to you in previous positions. For example in 3 the abdominal muscles can quake, 4 and 5 may make the thighs tremble and in 7 the legs can shake. The best way to counteract these sometimes forceful limb jerks is to keep pushing beyond them, keep stretching and breathing as slowly as you can. The good news is that this shows you are working the muscles, even if it feels unstable, twisted and uncontrollable. The shaking will eventually stop. You will notice you have more flexibility in your legs, your hamstrings will begin to lengthen and increase the mobility of your hips, pelvis and spine. This will in turn help you to perform the other positions. As I have said, each position helps with the development of the others.

I have been practising Kum Nye, daily, for over ten years. Some days the positions are liberating and flow with ease, other days they are incredibly challenging. If I am ever in doubt of what I am trying to achieve, all I need to do is remind myself of some of the people I have introduced Kum Nye to and remember their experiences and awakenings.

Karen is a good example. Karen attended one of my nine-week courses, attracted to the idea of a twenty-minute workout that would fit into her busy schedule. She was a self-employed therapist but spent most of her week running from one clinic to another leaving her little time to spend with her family and friends. Even her two-year relationship had not progressed past the 'two nights a week' stage.

From the first class Karen experienced a wide

range of both physical and emotional reactions. It began with a spontaneous release of tears and gasping for air while in the first position. For the following couple of weeks Karen experienced deep exhaustion and simply could not run around in the way she was used to. Karen allowed herself to surrender a little and began to question why she was running around with so few eggs in half-filled baskets. By always travelling against the clock and worrying about being late for her clients she was no longer focusing on her work itself. She also began to question her relationship. At 33 years old Karen realised that her arrangement of convenience was no longer enough. This sudden dissatisfaction with her life as she knew it precipitated a flood of responses. Tears, tantrums, chest infections, pimples, sciatic episodes were amongst the list of symptoms that made her stop and reassess her priorities. Each week we would hear the latest instalment. The relationship faltered, a new position became available in a clinic that was going to provide all the support she required in her job and utilise all her skills. She even managed to move house having been unable to find something suitable for four months. With a mixture of relief and nervousness she continued on her path of reconstruction.

Karen's experiences since embarking on the Kum Nye were faster than the average but perhaps the timing was right for her. By the time we came to the last class she had rearranged her work, moved and began a new courtship – with her previous partner! But all that didn't compare to the biggest achievement Karen made. A few weeks later, before the first revision class, Karen came bustling up to me, excited and child-like and said, 'You'll never guess what I did at the weekend . . . I went and sat on the grass for a few hours, just mesmerised!' I can still see her face beaming.

Although this is an example of someone who went through some big life changes, it is not uncommon for students to experience some such transformation and reorganising of their lives when they begin Kum Nye. Things that no longer work for you become easier to recognise and let go of. Your values are reassessed and with that your goals and ambitions may change or be reaffirmed in a clearer light. By slowing down to appreciate the natural world around you, you can begin to flow with it. Listen to the seasons, let your body tell you what foods you need to suit the changes in climate, or when you need more rest to boost your immune system to protect against winter coughs and colds.

While cycling around London, when the traffic, noise, aggression and confusion become too overwhelming I sometimes just stop and look at the sky. As I gaze upwards its magnitude and vastness puts everything back into perspective. Even on cloudy days I know the sun is shining above. The city becomes a façade compared to the complexities of the existence beyond it. The aggression and anxiety that are bounced from person to person like a live grenade lose their value and are dispersed into the vastness of space. The cacophony of sirens and vehicles begin to harmonise and blend together with a higher symphony. The numbers of birds become more noticeable and reclaim the sky from the vast aeroplane tracks. I feel light in my heart and continue on my journey.

Completing the cycle

Now that you have stretched and stretched again, here is how you finish. As you release your hands from your feet, rub your legs all over, as hard as you can. They have – hopefully – been stretched extensively and the rubbing will help to avoid any cramping or muscle tenderness and encourage circulation. When done, bring your legs down and roll onto your left side. Rest and breathe slowly to slow down your heart rate. Feel your muscles relaxing and easing and filling with revitalised energy, rested and restored.

Congratulations! You have just completed a full cycle of Kum Nye.

When you are ready, slowly rise. You are invigorated and awake, ready to start your day with a clear mind, body and soul.

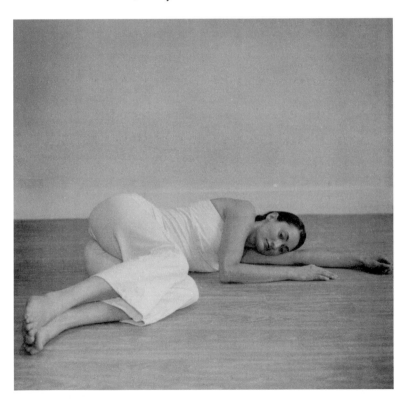

CHAPTER 9

Finding My Way with Kum Nye

I came across Tibetan Dur Bön medicine, and with it Kum Nye, by chance. Some would call it fate or destiny. Whatever it was, it became the most auspicious occurrence in my life so far.

Generally life was relatively uneventful. I plodded along, meandering past dozens of opportunities. There were a couple of incidents where I thanked my lucky stars that 'circumstances' allowed me to choose one course of action versus another and consequently prevented potentially disastrous outcomes. But on the whole I have played it relatively safe throughout my life. However, I wasn't particularly 'content' and was always looking for something, never completely satisfied. If something made me feel good I wanted more, but there was always a price to pay. The highs were never quite high enough but the lows seemed relentless. As a child, growing up in a small country town my most profound memory is of feeling discontented and isolated from the rest of the world. My escape was listening to music on FM radio. I was unable to find expression for my frustration, or able to grasp what the underlying cause of this inner turmoil was. I thought it was about being 'misunderstood'. Hindsight enables me to see it was also about 'misunderstanding'.

I eventually left New Zealand for Australia

to study Chiropractic. It was over the next ten years that I endeavoured to satisfy this 'desire without a name' that gnawed at my insides, confusing my emotions, clouding my judgement and lowering my vitality. I was working hard and playing hard yet still carrying that feeling of 'discontent'.

After ten years I decided to move again – this time to London. If arriving in Dalston isn't a reality check I don't know what is!

Finding an appropriate niche in a vast city is even more difficult. The job I had prearranged fell through, my relationship faltered and I found myself homeless. Then, at a fortuitous dinner party, I found myself talking to a friend of a friend. He mentioned that a friend of his knew someone who was setting up a clinic and was looking for complementary medicine practitioners to join. I said 'sure' and thought nothing of it. However, a few days later I found myself on the way to an appointment to meet Christopher Hansard.

Not long after, I was offered a job working at the clinic part time, which I accepted immediately.

During the third year of my Chiropractic degree I was introduced to Chinese medicine. I was so impressed by its effectiveness that I planned to study Chinese medicine once I had qualified and settled into the Chiropractic profession. I had looked at various courses but never quite found what I was looking for. Six months into working at Eden Medical Centre Christopher began to teach a small group of students who were interested in Tibetan medicine. Most were attracted to the spiritual nature of the teachings, while I was adamant I was only interested in learning the acupuncture – as an Eastern 'medical' system which I could study like a map of the body. With my Chiropractic knowledge I could comprehend how it worked in conjunction with the nervous system and certain Western models of anatomy and physiology. The spiritual stuff I was wary of. 'Energetics' were not my thing.

A few months on, I experienced a personal crisis and became overwrought. Christopher, seeing my distress, asked if I would allow him to help me and swiftly and skilfully he placed an acupuncture needle onto my head. I felt an intense wave of compassion, like a bolt of light exploding throughout my being and beyond. I can still feel it today. I knew then that this was the knowledge I wanted to harness, this was what I had been looking for, this was the experience I wanted to understand.

———

Through my daily meditations and Kum Nye practice, slowly, bit by bit the sun began to shine through the clouds in my mind. I spontaneously began to experience happiness and joy, not all at once, just little glimpses that grew and grew.

My senses were improving and my dreams became more vivid. My body continued to get stronger. Physically I had experienced a total systems purge, inside out.

To begin with I found these changes a little overwhelming and whenever the boundaries of my everyday realities became challenged I would panic and retreat. But Kum Nye is about having the courage to know and accept yourself without judgement and I began to experience being in my heart.

As part of my training in Tibetan Dur Bön medicine I am required to undertake various retreats. A retreat is designed to allow you to gain spiritual knowledge, to become more aware, awakened, balanced and insightful and at peace with your life.

Becoming 'one with the universe' is all very noble but there are usually some personal prejudices, denials and defences to deal with along the way and in order to sustain this connectedness you have to be willing to really see yourself – warts and all. We all hold positive and negative emotions within ourselves. The trick is to view each negative emotion as a teacher we can learn from. We would not be human if we did not experience the whole gamut of emotions, even though at times we may deny that we do. We grow spiritually and emotionally when we learn to understand how these emotions affect ourselves and other people around us. Think how anger spreads from one person to another. Recognising your own patterns and the origins of these patterns liberates you. Acknowledging and accepting who you are, what influenced your development and how this evolved, enables you to move forward. This is tough work and only you can do it for yourself.

A retreat can be performed anywhere. I had it lucky! My first retreat was performed in a warm, secure and comfortable apartment on the coast of Cornwall for nine days over Christmas and New Year. I had no contact with the outside world except for watching the winter skies and raging seas through the double-glazed windows. I felt encapsulated from the world. As a holiday home it would have been pure luxury but as a retreat, it felt like an isolation chamber.

While the world outside overindulged in

seasonal festivities I would begin each day with my meditations and Kum Nye, then sit drumming and chanting. Each day brought a gamut of emotions and frustrations as I struggled to persevere with this seemingly easy regime. Increasingly, my Kum Nye practice became stronger and more enjoyable as I slowly became clearer, while the chanting and drumming cleansed my body, mind and spirit.

One night, after finishing for the day, I lay on the floor, my body buzzing with vibrations which began to intensify until they became what I can only describe as a clear light.

I lay there for hours feeling my heart open and bloom, connecting my mind, body and spirit as the sensations coursed through me. The next day I discovered that Position 5, Honour to the Earth King had shifted. The position produced the most intense heat that travelled from my chest down my arms to my hands and beyond. The position felt strong, vibrant and liberating. I was elated and energised and very excited at the realisation of what I had experienced.

Over the next few months, one by one, each position began to shift and change and I began to gain new perspectives of various little, yet important, aspects of my life and settled into a broader awareness of both my environment and my relationships within it.

While these insights can occur at any time throughout one's life and are not specific to Kum Nye, the practise does give rise to these types of experiences. Kum Nye remains an enigma, one I hope you will enjoy and gain personal wisdom from, as I too continue to do. This is just the beginning.

———

APPENDIX

To help you understand the variety of mystical, emotional and spiritual aspects of Kum Nye I am including a few case histories that some of the students have been generous enough to permit my using.

David came to the Eden Medical Centre to see Christopher Hansard, my teacher, with high blood pressure. For his particular condition and the underlying nature of his illness, the main part of his treatment programme was to be the

Kum Nye. Initially I started David on an intense programme concentrating on the first three positions for a few months until his cardio-vascular system began to strengthen. He then incorporated the rest of the positions to maintain the balance of all his body's systems, structural, physiological and psychological.

This is how David explains his experience of Kum Nye: 'Kum Nye seemed at first some sort of indulgence that I must do to satisfy Christopher Hansard in his prescribed treatment of my high blood pressure. The first few sessions were very uncomfortable even though I am quite limber and not unaccustomed to yoga or Pilates. At one point, during the introduction of the sixth position where one squats with hands folded there was acute pain to my knees. Having previously, several years ago, torn my anterior cruciate ligament with subsequent rehabilitation where the therapist warned me of overextending the joint, I was fearful of pushing through the pain to accomplish the exercise. Your insistence that it would be OK somehow encouraged me to work through the pain, breathe and see what happened. Today, as a result of success with this particular exercise I ski without fear of hyperextending my knees. I now look forward to staying in this position for extended periods because it feels so good.

'At some point during the sequence of postures a strange sound emerged in my ears; a kind of white sound that seemed to float me in a sort of trance state.

'Even during the more difficult positions I can just watch my body as it holds and breathes, there is an ethereal quality to the whole session.

———

'The days that I practise as opposed to those days that I do not are qualitatively different, fuller and seemingly more complete as I approach the day.

'Kum Nye has produced wealth, love and success in huge quantities in my life. In fact during the standing position when my arms are extended to the sky I envision clearing my space to receive richness. I have nicknamed this exercise "Yes, I am open to more". No, I have not won the lottery. I have not turned back the clock thirty years nor have I been discovered by Hollywood. But Kum Nye has somehow allowed a huge shift in my day to welcome more of the moment and appreciate the fullness thereof.'

Ellen explains how she came to discover the effects and benefits of Kum Nye. She experienced things very quickly when she began Kum Nye. I have included this testament to give you an example of what it is possible to encounter. I must stress that not all people experience such an array of effects, nor so quickly.

'I started my journey with Kum Nye in August 2002 after reading about it in a local magazine. It immediately struck a chord with me. I liked the idea that it was energising, needed little space, no special equipment and it was only twenty minutes each morning.

'I started and struggled through the first few weeks of lessons and new movements. After about a month I had learned four of the eight movements and was finding that each morning as I worked on the movement I felt a strong sense of rightness of the situation. I also found some odd things were beginning to happen. I felt ravenous for most of the first few weeks, craving things I don't normally like, such as a steak. This passed after about six weeks and then my appetite actually decreased from its original level.

'In terms of the movements I suddenly found that the second position was becoming impossible to hold and that was a struggle for several weeks. Meanwhile I found the whole concept of 'breath' difficult – the combination of strong movements and breathing was tough. The breath would stick in my solar plexus and it was hard to make it move down through the rest of my body.

'After a few weeks I was able to hold the second movement but began to have real issues with the third. I have finally worked through this and now after a full seven months of Kum

Nye, I make a long, loud noise with the breath in this movement. It is like a long AHHHHHH sound. It feels wonderful – like a strong release of tension. It feels cleansing and energising at the same time.

'One of the fascinating things about my Kum Nye experience is the many different effects it has had on my body. In the beginning I was rife with "gas" that seemed to coincide with the ravenous hunger – when that lifted, so did the gas problem. I have always struggled with irritable bowel syndrome and have found the Kum Nye has dramatically improved this problem and my abdominal swelling and pain has mostly gone now!

'Aside from the physical changes there were emotional issues at play as well. I started Kum Nye at a very important moment in my career.

———

I was feeling down, seriously contemplating leaving my job and knowing that a major change was needed in my life. I quit my job six weeks into the Kum Nye and felt the most unbelievable sense of lightness and rightness with this decision. About the same time I found I moved to another level with the Kum Nye, thus finding that as my emotions moved so did my ability to move that small next step with my Kum Nye.

'I started a course which I was hoping would be the key to my new career developments. The course was a catastrophe, I struggled with it and in the middle of this my computer crashed losing all of my data. It was as if the fates were telling me to throw out the old life. I cleaned the cupboards and purged years of paper. I shrugged off losing the data with remarkable calm – it sort of felt right. But I was deeply panicked and unsure about the future. I was again struggling with Kum Nye every morning and just could not seem to push myself to improve.

'While on holiday I began to see the way forward in my career. I made strong, bold decisions. I decided I would not go back to school or get a job working for some company. I would look to find a business to buy.

'Upon returning to London with this plan of action, I felt lighter and happier than I had in years. It was like I could feel "Ellen" returning. My first day back I woke up early and nervously attempted Kum Nye. It was a miracle — I had moved forward here as well. Suddenly the movements were flowing again and especially the breath — it was all new and much easier.'

Ann-Louise had this to say about Kum Nye: 'It has been a complete joy to learn the art of Kum Nye. I fully accept and respect this wonderful set of eight exercises as my daily spiritual discipline that balances and energises me holistically, enabling me to be more focused for the day to come.

'Whilst practising Kum Nye I find myself shut off from the "outside material" world and I have entered the "inner spiritual" world where I find the peace and calm I crave, giving me answers and messages to many questions.

'Kum Nye is the spiritual nourishment that is as important to me as eating my breakfast every morning; creating reserves of strength mentally, emotionally and physically. Paranoias are slowly dissolving. I have been going round and round in circles for some time now trying to find my path. Kum Nye has been a big milestone on this spiritual journey and is straightening the road for me.'

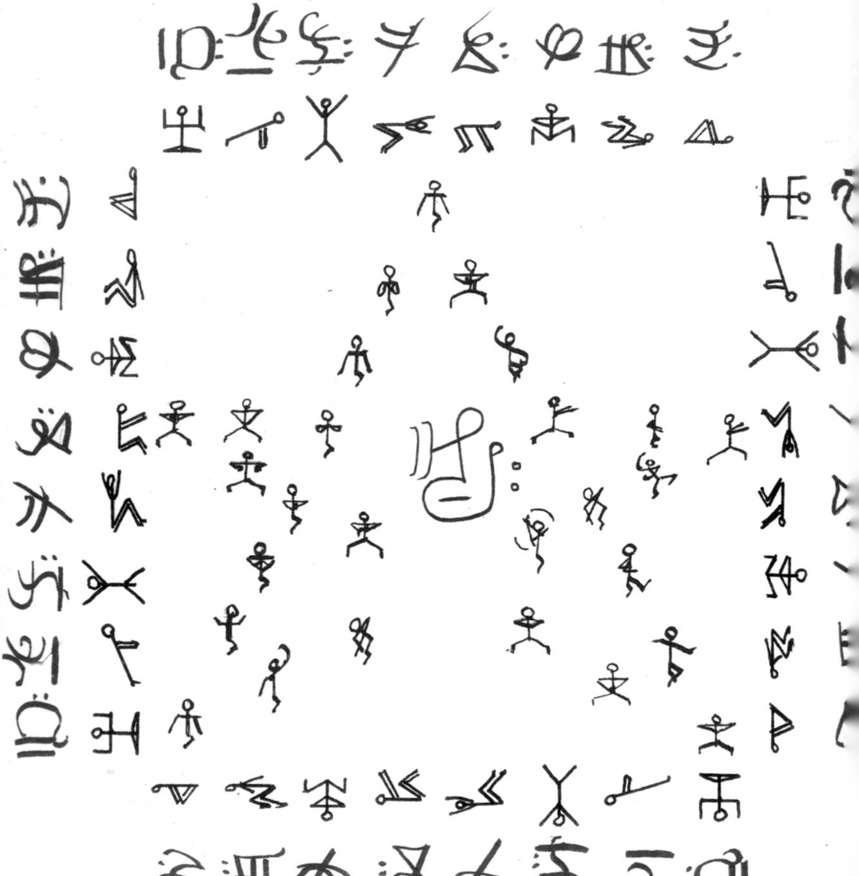